# JOSHUA'S JOURNEY

## One Boy's Victory Over Allergies

SALLY JADLOW

ISBN-13: 978-1724882424

ISBN-10: 1724882422

Cover design by MJ Freeman of Valiant Courier Publications

# DEDICATION

This book is dedicated to the One who sees, hears, and answers prayer.

# Table of Contents


Joshua's Beginnings ..... 1

Additional Problems ..... 3

A Teacher's Request ..... 7

A Breakthrough ..... 9

The Phil Donahue Show ..... 11

Grand Mal Seizure ..... 13

Dr. Rapp's Book ..... 15

A Fly in the Ointment ..... 19

Our Appointment ..... 21

The Results ..... 25

For Further Information ..... 31

*Sally Jadlow*

# Joshua's Beginnings

Our fourth child was definitely different from the others. By eighteen months we discovered Josh couldn't see things near him. Instead of picking at small objects on the floor as most children do, he preferred to climb the kitchen cabinets to reach the stemmed glassware on the top shelves. After an eye doctor appointment, we learned he was extremely far sighted. The muscle in one eye didn't keep a constant tension. When he tried to walk, he'd take a few steps, then fall. He'd get up and try again. My heart broke to watch him struggle.

A few months later, surgery helped correct that muscle problem. In addition, the doctors fitted him with tiny glasses to strengthen his eye muscle. When we walked hand-in-hand out of the eye doctor's office the day he got his glasses, Josh paused, bent down, and felt blades of grass he'd never seen clearly. With wonder in his voice he said, "Grass."

I put him in his car seat and headed for home. He screamed and cried and pulled at his glasses. He'd never been able to see objects flying past the car windows. It took a couple of weeks for him to adjust to his new-found sight.

When he was two and a half at his regular eye appointment, the doctor discovered Josh had developed cataracts. Within a year he underwent cataract surgery in each eye.

The doctor said they couldn't insert lens implants because his eyeballs would grow. Josh would have to wait several years for ocular implants. He had to wear big thick glasses that were set at +23 power. This made him appear bug-eyed. Most children were afraid of him. I was extremely distressed each time I saw one of them mistreat him.

The weight of his glasses caused them to come off easily. I sewed bands of elastic to go around the back and over the top of his head. This made him even more conspicuous.

# Additional Problems

I shuddered as four-year-old Josh let loose with another earsplitting scream. He sat glued to the TV. Would he ever quit with this irritation? I rounded the corner into the family room. He seemed engrossed in silly cartoons playing on the screen. Nothing scary there. Josh seemed to be unaware of his habit. What made him do this?

Josh did another thing that nearly drove me crazy. He'd unconsciously chew on his collar while he watched TV. I looked through his closet one day and discovered he didn't have one decent shirt to wear. Was he hungry? Anxious? Bored? Why would anyone chew their clothes like this?

Before he entered kindergarten at age five, the school wanted to have him take an IQ test to know where to place him. The teachers had my husband, Vic, and I meet with them to learn the results of the test. The report came back with an IQ of 53.

Fifty-three? Were they serious? I didn't want to question their assessment, so I politely replied, "I'm not too sure your test is correct."

Later in the conversation, I commented on his extreme helpfulness. "He loves to unload the dishwasher and put the silverware away."

One of the teachers sat forward, "Really? He can sort silverware?"

"Yes. Why?"

"Most children with an IQ that low can't manage a task like sorting silverware."

Now I was even more convinced the tests were wrong. I made our dilemma an object of prayer.

The school labeled him "Special Ed" and placed him in a small classroom with a handful of other students with special needs.

The next year when it was time for his IEP evaluation we met with the teachers again. At the end of the meeting I asked, "What do you envision for Josh, long term?"

The teachers shifted and glanced at one another. Finally, one spoke. "Josh might be able to live in a group home one day. He might even be able to have a little job like stuffing envelopes."

On the way home, Vic refused to talk about the teachers' assessment.

I, on the other hand, didn't remain silent. "Those people are wrong! Josh has a brighter future than that. There's more in that brain than what their tests show."

Continuing to pray, I sought the Lord Jesus for answers. In addition to his high-pitched screams, he sometimes jerked involuntarily and had episodes of rapid hand clapping. At times he would stiffen his fingers, pull in his chin, and roll his eyes up. Sometimes Josh chewed his knuckles. Perhaps those manifestations were from something like Tourette's Syndrome.

We took Josh to a pediatric neurologist at Children's Mercy Hospital. After a thorough examination, the doctor concluded Josh didn't have Tourette's, but he failed to come up with any other diagnosis.

At times Josh's skin itched and his hands swelled. Sometimes he found it impossible to concentrate. He also had little small muscle control. Doctors didn't have any solutions for those symptoms either. Whatever was wrong also affected his bowels and caused him to have headaches. He frequently experienced abdominal pains, gas, belching, and diarrhea. Very seldom did he have a dry bed at night.

When we ate out, Josh frequently rubbed his head on the booth. At school, he had little comprehension when reading because he'd skip lines.

One summer day after Josh ate peanut butter, I gave him chalk to draw on the sidewalk. He happily went outside and printed his letters and his name backward. That seemed strange. If he were dyslexic wouldn't he write backwards all the time? What made him react this way?

It seemed the more I prayed, the more symptoms our son exhibited. There had to be an answer to all this weird behavior—but what was it? How would I find out?

# A Teacher's Request

His first-grade teacher suggested we might look into the possibility of contact lenses instead of the thick glasses that made him appear bug-eyed. Josh discovered he could scare the other children by pretending to be a monster when they teased him. The teacher didn't appreciate the constant disruption.

When we asked the pediatric ophthalmologist about that idea he flatly refused.

"He's too young. He'll lose them often. They aren't covered by insurance."

In spite of his thick glasses, I signed him up for softball the summer after his first-grade year. Maybe sports would help him interact better with other children.

The boys on the team promptly rejected him. Josh's hand-eye coordination was extremely slow. The ball was long past the bat by the time he swung.

On the way home after practice one day Josh said, "I don't want to play softball anymore."

"Why son? Don't you enjoy it?"

"I can't hit the ball."

"Well, with some more practice you'll get better."

Josh sat silent for several blocks, then said, "When I went up to bat today some of the boys spit on me."

"Did the coach see it?"

"I don't know. He didn't say anything."

I took him off the team immediately. We'd have to find another activity for this little one.

# A Breakthrough

One weekend our family went to Truman Lake in southern Missouri. A couple across the room in a small restaurant seemed very interested in Josh. Finally, the wife approached us.

"Has your son had cataract surgery?"

I answered, "Yes. Why?"

"Our son had to wear those big thick glasses after his surgery. He's about your son's age. He wears contacts now."

As we visited, we learned they were from the Kansas City area and had previously gone to the same pediatric ophthalmologist Josh currently saw.

She said, "We switched to another doctor after the first one refused to prescribe contacts."

I quickly jotted down the name of their current doctor. At home, I made an appointment for Josh with the new doctor. Within two weeks after seeing this second doctor, Josh had new contacts. They were very thick—+23 power. Each one cost $250.00. The doctor let us know that was his cost price; that he wasn't making a dime.

These contacts only had to be taken out and cleaned once a week.

The first doctor was right. Josh frequently lost one, especially if he rubbed his eyes.

When he'd lose one, we'd go on a mad-dash hunt to look for it. Sometimes I'd find it in the side of his waterbed. Other times we'd find it on the carpet.

I'd ask, "Josh, don't you get a headache when you lose one?"

He'd shake his head.

If it hadn't been out too long, I could sometimes put it in the cleaning solution to rehydrate it. Other times we'd be looking at another $250-dollar bill. Even though the expense was heavy, it was worth it because people's reaction to him was entirely different.

# **The Phil Donahue Show**

My cousin called one day. "Are you watching the Phil Donahue Show? There's a kid on there that sounds like Josh."

I flipped on the TV. Phil interviewed a young boy who suffered allergies to everything.

At one point in the show the boy requested, "Could you please remove the person wearing perfume? Perfume makes me want to kiss people."

To most people that would sound like a silly request, but immediately I remembered a Christmas pageant years earlier at church. Chuckles rippled across the audience as Josh kept trying to kiss the little girl next to him. Although the audience found it entertaining, I didn't. If I could have gotten him off the stage somehow, I would have—but of course that was impossible.

Another instance came to mind. Our neighbor always wore perfume. When her granddaughter visited from out of state our family joined them on the patio for dinner. Josh chased her around the yard with the intent to kiss her also.

Could he be allergic to perfume? Maybe there was something to what this kid said. Maybe this program held answers to Joshua's problems. I sat to listen.

After the set was cleared of the perfume scent, Phil introduced the young boy's allergy doctor, Dr. Doris Rapp. She had written a book, *Is This Your Child?*

During the interview Dr. Rapp shared how she practiced a different method of testing called Provocation Neutralization. Instead of making scratches all over a patient's back to determine what they were allergic to, she administered a series of injections of one irritant at a time. Then she had the child's parent observe their child and note any reactions.

This method sounded interesting, but she was located somewhere in New York. I knew the chances were slim we'd ever make that kind of trip.

The next Sunday at church I asked an allergist I knew, "Do you think allergies could cause bizarre behavior?"

"Oh no. That's ridiculous. Allergies don't affect behavior."

I wasn't so sure, especially after what I'd seen on the Donahue show.

That next week I hunted until I found an allergist in Kansas City who tested patients with the Provocation Neutralization method Dr. Rapp mentioned and made an appointment.

After testing, we learned Josh was allergic to eggs, milk, corn, sugar, wheat, soy, yeast, and peanut butter. Although I wanted the doctor to test him further, he was not equipped to test for more.

Little could be done for Josh, so I avoided feeding him the offending foods as much as possible. He continued with his weird habits.

What else was he allergic to? Maybe with any luck, he'd outgrow these allergies.

# Grand Mal Seizure

The special education teachers in second grade reported Josh had a terrible time retaining what he was taught. His handwriting was illegible. Josh frequently wet his pants, although he had been trained since he was two. Sometimes he lost control of his bowels. The teacher kept an extra set of clothes at school for him. At times, I'd receive a call to bring a fresh set before the day was over.

Since his printing was usually not decipherable, the teachers decided he needed to learn to type. It took him a year and a half before he mastered the keyboard.

Everything he attempted seemed a monumental effort. I marveled at his attitude through it all. When he'd fail at a task he'd smile and say, "I'll try again." Eventually, he'd succeed and move on to learning a new skill.

By the end of third grade, the teacher suggested they hold him back a year because of his slow progress. "Better now than later," she said.

With heavy hearts, we agreed.

At the end of that next school year his teacher received a new desk in their small closed special ed classroom. The teacher seated Josh next to the plastic desk.

That afternoon I got a call from her. In a rather tense tone she said, "Mrs. Jadlow, you need to come pick up Josh."

I couldn't read her tone. Was she angry? "Has he had another accident? Didn't he still have an extra set of clothes at school?"

The teacher sighed. "It's not that. He's had a grand mal seizure."

"What? He's never had one before. Are you sure? Maybe it was only a petite mal."

"I'm sure. In my off hours I'm an Emergency Medical Technician. I've witnessed this before. I know a grand mal when I see one. You need to ask the doctor to order an electroencephalogram (EEG). That might show if there is brain damage."

"Oh," was all I could choke out. What were we going to do? Not only were my hopes he'd outgrow these troubles dashed, now they seemed to be multiplying.

Josh and I went through the motions to get the EEG as the teacher advised. It came back negative. Now what?

# Dr. Rapp's Book

The last day of school of his second time through third grade the teacher took the class to a park for a picnic. When Josh came in the door that afternoon he burst into tears, let loose with a tirade, and ran to his room. He said he hated me.

This unbelievable behavior went on for over four hours. I couldn't get any rational word from him.

Finally, the sobbing stopped. I headed for his room and met him in the hall. He hugged me and between gasps he said, "Mom, I'm sorry. I didn't mean those things. I don't know what made me say that stuff. I couldn't stop crying."

With further questioning I learned he drank a common lemon/lime cola at the picnic. Maybe there was something in that drink that caused this horrible reaction. I made a mental note—no more of that drink— ever.

During the summer of his tenth year my frustration grew with each pair of messy pants. With one hand holding his underpants in the toilet and the other on the flush handle I screamed, "I can't take this anymore!"

The doctor's interview on Donahue came to mind. Perhaps Dr. Rapp's book might have some answers. I bought it and began to read. As

I devoured page after page, my hope grew that maybe this woman's practice held the key to our dilemma.

Since I could not locate a doctor in this area who practiced Dr. Rapp's extensive method of testing, we'd have to go to New York. The thought of navigating New York City paralyzed me.

Flipping to the back of the book I saw Dr. Rapp wasn't in New York City after all. She practiced in Buffalo, New York! Why had I not noticed this before? This changed everything. I continued to read Dr. Rapp's book with new eyes.

She gave very strict steps a patient had to accomplish before she would consider seeing them in her office.

The first requirement—an elimination diet. (Food Elimination Diets can be found on page 171 of Dr. Rapp's book, *Is This Your Child?*)

For the first day, the patient eats nothing but soda crackers. Then one new food is introduced each day. The parent is to note if they observe any reaction in their child such as aggressive behavior, if the child develops circles under his eyes, has red cheeks or ears, or has a lack of attention, is unable to write legibly, or has a change in attitude when the new food is introduced.

When we began the elimination diet, I noticed Josh wrote much more legibly and had fewer weird noises while watching TV. During that first week his diet consisted of oatmeal with honey for breakfast, a beef or chicken vegetable soup with a rice cake and a banana for lunch, and some form of chicken breast with fresh vegetable, potato and fresh salad for dinner with water. I noted during that week he stopped chewing his knuckles.

The second week we began to add dairy products. That first lunch he ate milk, white cheese, cottage cheese and uncolored butter. Within 10 minutes he stiffened his fingers and pulled in his chin and rolled his eyes up. In the afternoon he became argumentative. At dinner we went out to eat. He ate half an eight-ounce steak and a half of a baked potato with sour cream and butter. Within ten minutes he seemed to lose concentration and didn't finish his dinner. He rubbed his head on the back of the booth and said he was tired.

The next day he had wet pants and messed them also. We added flour to the diet that day. The teacher said he had trouble concentrating and skipped lines when he tried to read. He had to point to each word in order to read at all. In the evening, he didn't want to work on learning the keyboard. Instead he cut up paper into tiny pieces.

When we added sugar, he wasn't able to write as well and wet his bed at night. On adding chocolate, he filled his pants, had a headache, made weird movements with his hands, and had a wet bed the next morning.

We stuck with the diet until we'd finished. By then, I had a pretty good handle on the things Dr. Rapp needed to test for.

I sent Josh's charted reactions to Dr. Rapp's office. The staff sent a thick packet of questions. These questions covered not only the suspected irritants, but also the patient's reactions.

In the packet, Dr. Rapp asked many details about Josh's life such as what kind of house he lived in. Was the garage attached? What is the current mold counts in the atmosphere? I had to check with Children's Mercy Hospital for that one. The questions seemed endless.

With the paperwork finished, I called Dr. Rapp's office in early September to set an appointment. We were scheduled for early November and made our airline reservations. This was really happening. Oh, how I hoped this trip was not in vain.

During the fall the doctor's office sent a kit to test the air at school, church, and home. I opened the shipping box and found a plastic file box inside equipped with an aquarium bubbler to oxygenate water. I was to put distilled water in a pint jar and set the bubbler to cycle the water for several hours in each place Josh spent time. Each place used a fresh pint of water.

Before we left, I was instructed to send the whole kit back with the jars labeled "home air," "school air," and "church air." The doctor planned to use a distillation of this fluid in her testing procedure.

I finished all the instructions and sent the water back to Buffalo. One more step accomplished.

# A Fly in the Ointment

A week before we were to leave, Dr. Rapp's office called. The nurse informed me the doctor would not see Josh.

My heart skipped a beat. "Why not? We've done all the required testing. We have our airline tickets and motel reservations. What did we do wrong?"

"You didn't do anything wrong. When we went through the papers you sent back, we saw Josh had a grand mal seizure. It's our policy not to allow children with seizure disorders to be tested in the office. If he experienced one here, he might scare the other children undergoing testing. You see, all the children are tested together in one big room."

"But that was only one time. It was after the teacher got a new plastic desk. He's not had another."

All our work and planning was down the drain. Where would we go from here? Did they not understand what we'd been through? The indignities Josh had suffered for ten years?

All my frustrations came out like a bursting dam. "You can't do this to us! We've been through too much to be turned away. He needs Dr. Rapp's help. Don't you understand? There's no one in Kansas City to do this kind of testing."

The voice on the other end said, "We can check with the doctor and get back with you."

"Please do," was all I could manage.

I dissolved into a puddle, crying out to the Lord.

Within the hour the office employee called back. "Mrs. Jadlow, Dr. Rapp agreed to see him since the seizure had been a one-time episode."

A heavy weight lifted from my shoulders. I could breathe again. "Thank you! Oh, thank you."

The next week we were at the airport with hearts full of hope, ready for answers.

On the flight there, my seat-mate learned we intended to stay a week in Buffalo. "Oh, I hope you don't get too much snow. November in Buffalo can be pretty wicked."

I prayed a silent prayer we'd be spared bad weather. Before the week was out, I heard many comments from residents about the lack of snow.

# Our Appointment

Josh and I flew in a day early. Since we had the day free, we decided to play tourist and visit Niagara Falls and Fort Niagara. By evening we stopped at a quaint little restaurant for dinner. Before our meal came, Josh rested his head on his arm at the table. He fell asleep immediately. He'd never done this before. I sighed. Maybe by week's end we'd have some answers to a multitude of questions.

The next morning, we met with Dr. Rapp. After a short interview she showed us into a large room. Children lined the walls. Each child received an injection every five minutes of suspected allergens. Their parents sat nearby to chart any reactions.

Dr. Rapp explained, "When you go home, you'll be able to recognize the offending substance. Then you can remove him from it. We'll also send you home with a vial of Benadryl to give him in order to stop a reaction."

I seated myself, pen in hand and looked around the room, there were children from all parts of the nation and around the world.

One little boy from Israel exhibited a violent reaction to chicken. I later learned his family served meat only once a week—chicken—which was the very thing he was allergic to.

The doctor instructed the child next to us to remove his shoes. I asked the doctor, "Should Josh remove his?"

She shook her head and smiled.

The nurse injected him with a distillation of cat hair. Within five minutes the boy began to thrash about. He kicked the wall so hard the clock above me fell off and hit me on the head. So much for the Kansas City doctor's opinion that allergies don't alter behavior! I wondered if Josh would have such violent reactions.

Before Dr. Rapp injected Josh with school air she had him write his name. He stayed pretty much in the lines. With each injection at five-minute intervals his printing became more illegible until he could hardly fit a J on an entire sheet.

When they tested him with carpet glue the doctor videotaped him reading before any injections. He did fairly well. With each shot, reading became more difficult. After several doses he stared at the book a long while, gave the doctor a quizzical look and said, "I can't read this."

We discovered certain molds caused the high-pitched screams and caused him to chew his collar. Different spores caused him to fall asleep.

Doctor Rapp laughed when she learned we went to Niagara Falls the previous day. "That's the last place you should have been. That air is loaded with mold."

Sodium benzoate caused the uncontrolled crying. I was shocked to learn sodium benzoate is added to many foods as a preservative including popular lemon/lime drinks and even catsup.

By the end of the week we discovered Josh was allergic to many additives, preservatives, food colorings, school air, church air, and home air, peanut butter, petroleum-based products (plastics), mold, new carpet and carpet glue—to name a few.

No wonder he couldn't learn. His school was new and had carpet everywhere. This had been an eye-opening week for us. Hopefully we had found the answers we'd been searching for so long.

On our last day in Buffalo the nurses taught me how to give Josh shots. They sent us home with small vials of the offending substances with instructions to give him shots from each vial every day.

We received a food rotation diet that varied everything from cooking oils to vegetables, meats, and fruits. We would eat nothing from the same botanical food group more often than once every five days.

In her book *Is This Your Child?* Dr. Rapp gives a 4-day rotation diet on page 462.

# The Results

Back home at the beginning of his fourth-grade year, it was time for another IQ test. In a follow-up meeting with the teachers, they were puzzled at his score. It had jumped several points to 64.

"Who conducted the previous tests? Were they administered correctly?" his social worked asked. A teacher chimed in with, "This much of a point difference just doesn't happen."

As the teachers commented, I recalled his first IQ test. He sat on new carpet and the teacher fed him various colored candies as a reward. No wonder Josh came out with a low score!

I pictured his current classroom. New carpet not only covered the floor. To keep the noise levels low in the open concept design, they ran the carpet up those half-walls also.

Each day I diligently gave him shots of the things to which he was allergic, including small vials of the distilled water we had sent the doctor from his school, church, and home.

Eventually, we were able to reduce the shots to every other day, then every third day. By the end of the first year, Josh only received shots once a week.

We stayed on the strict rotation diet Dr. Rapp gave him for seven months.

After a year, Josh had no signs of allergy. He was able to learn and retain what he was taught. He scored a 78 when he took another IQ test at the beginning of his seventh-grade year.

Through his middle school and high school years Josh was on the honor roll every quarter.

The teachers quit giving him IQ tests in high school because on the last one he scored an 89. If he'd scored any higher, he would no longer meet the criteria for special education classes. The school would lose state funding for a special ed student. In their eyes, that would never do.

When Josh was sixteen, he got a part-time job cleaning churches after school. He worked hard in his Boy Scout troop and attained the rank of Eagle Scout. In addition, he earned three more merit badges after his Eagle award and received the Bronze Palm.

Today, Josh is a highly valued employee with a cleaning service. He has no reactions to any substances except to fresh asphalt. When his residential street was paved last year he looked like he had pink eye for about three days.

I often wonder what Josh's life would have been like had it not been for Dr. Rapp who fought for kids every day through her diligent practice.

The following pages are examples of Joshua's writing when being tested for various substances.

Several numbers are backwards.

| | | | | | |
|---|---|---|---|---|---|
| 11 | 12 | 13 | 14 | 15 | 16 |
| 21 | 22 | 23 | 24 | 25 | 56 |
| 13 | 35 | 33 | 34 | 35 | 36 |
| 41 | 45 | 43 | 41 | 45 | 46 |
| 61 | 55 | 53 | 55 | 54 | 56 |
| 61 | 65 | 63 | 66 | 65 | 66 |
| 71 | 75 | 73 | 74 | 75 | 76 |
| 81 | 82 | 83 | 84 | 85 | 86 |
| 41 | 42 | 93 | 44 | 95 | 96 |

I wrote a line then he wrote the next. This is after a week of being on the elimination diet before we started adding foods back in.

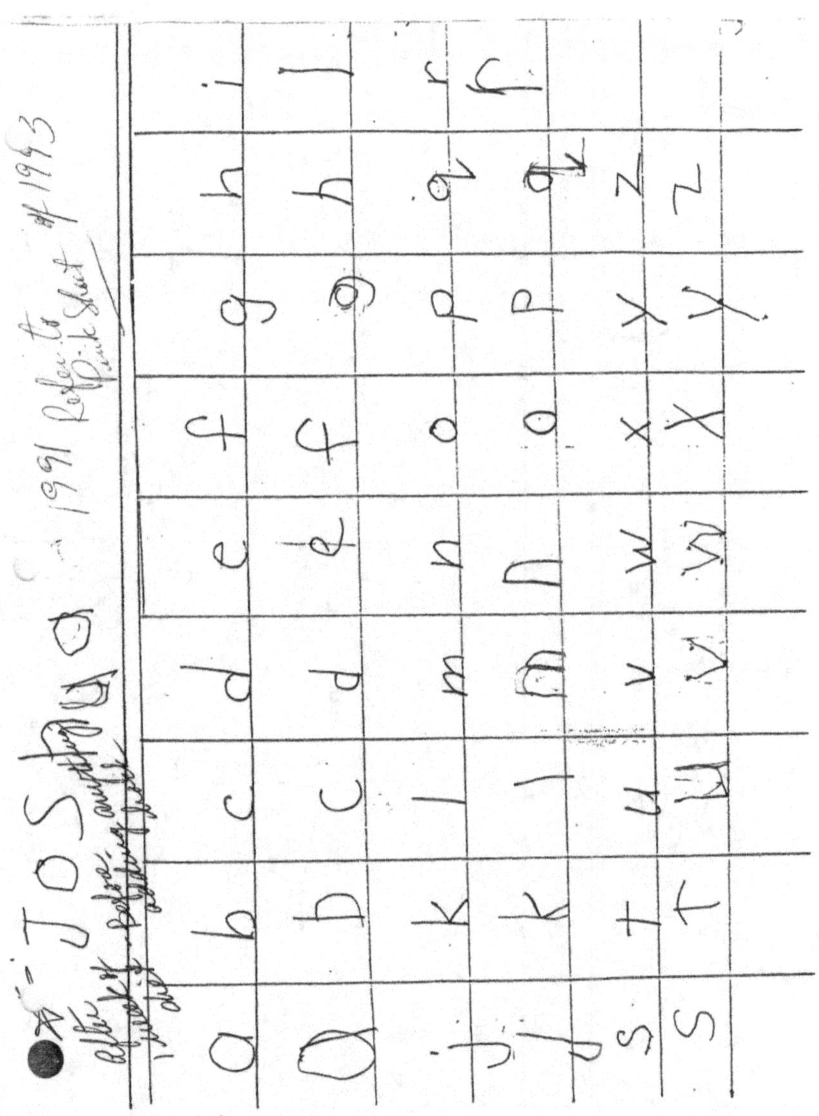

This is what Josh's name looked like when we tested for wheat.

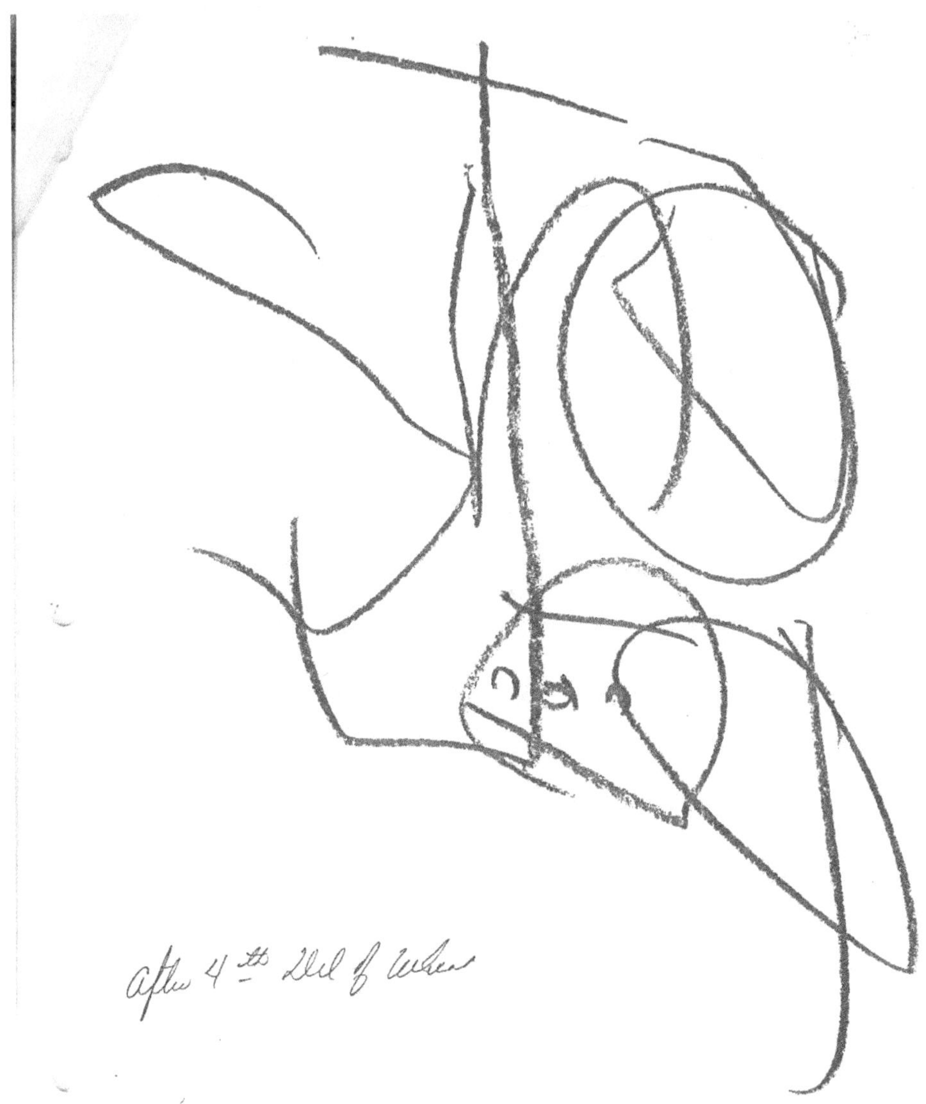

Evidently sugar was not a problem, but peanut butter was. His writing becomes completely backwards two hours after ingesting peanut butter.

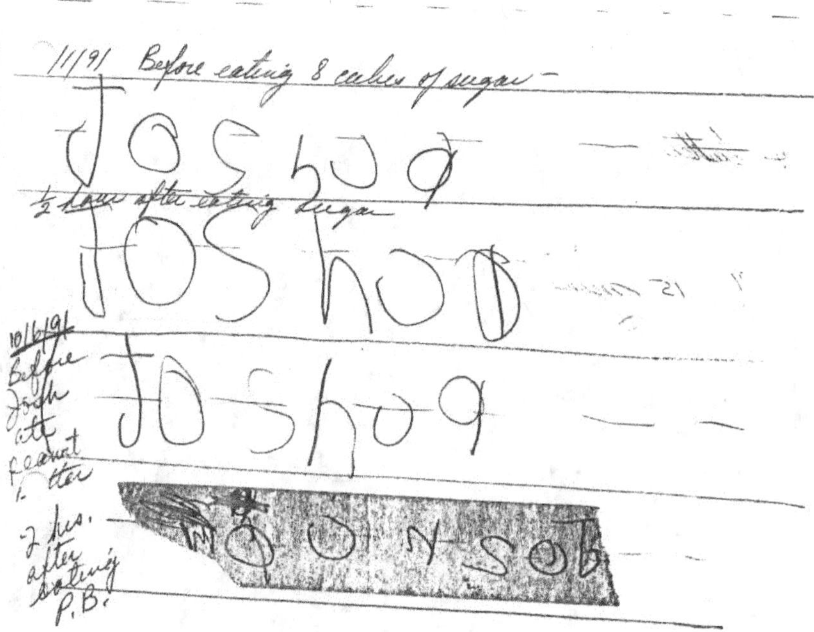

# For Further Information

For YouTube Videos:

https://www.youtube.com/watch?v=5pxeU_kHDFs

https://www.youtube.com/watch?v=hMKL8NF3I50

https://www.youtube.com/watch?v=dPo3Wi7Au7Y

Josh and Dr. Rapp in her office

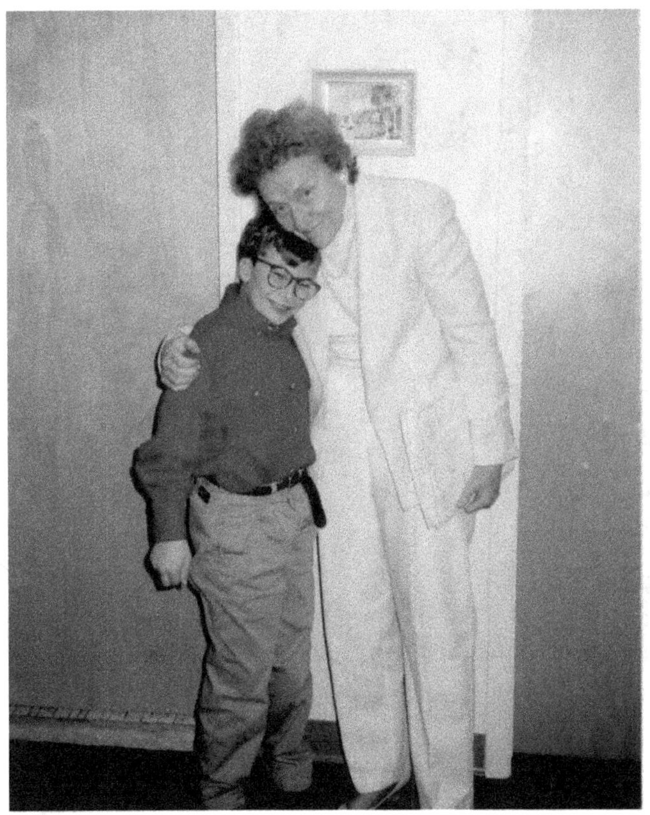

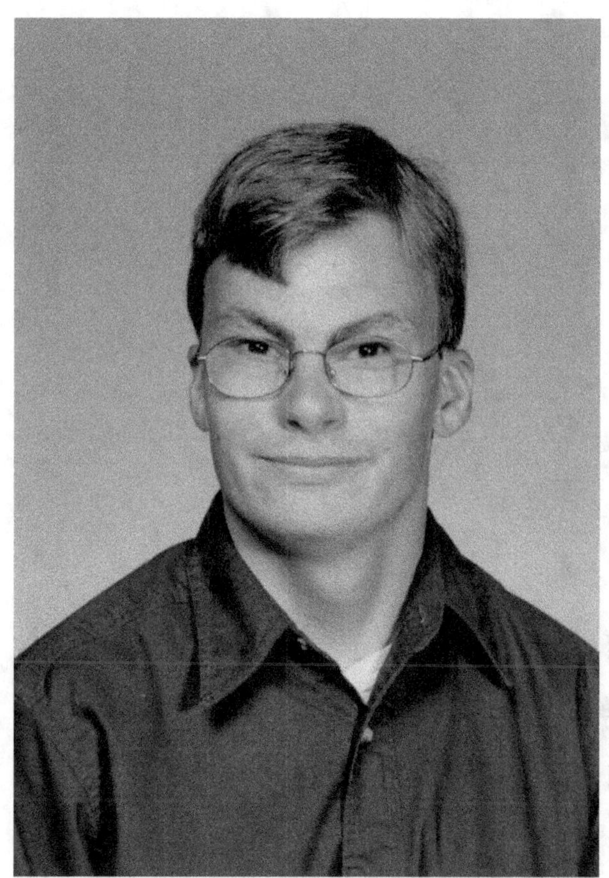

Josh in High School

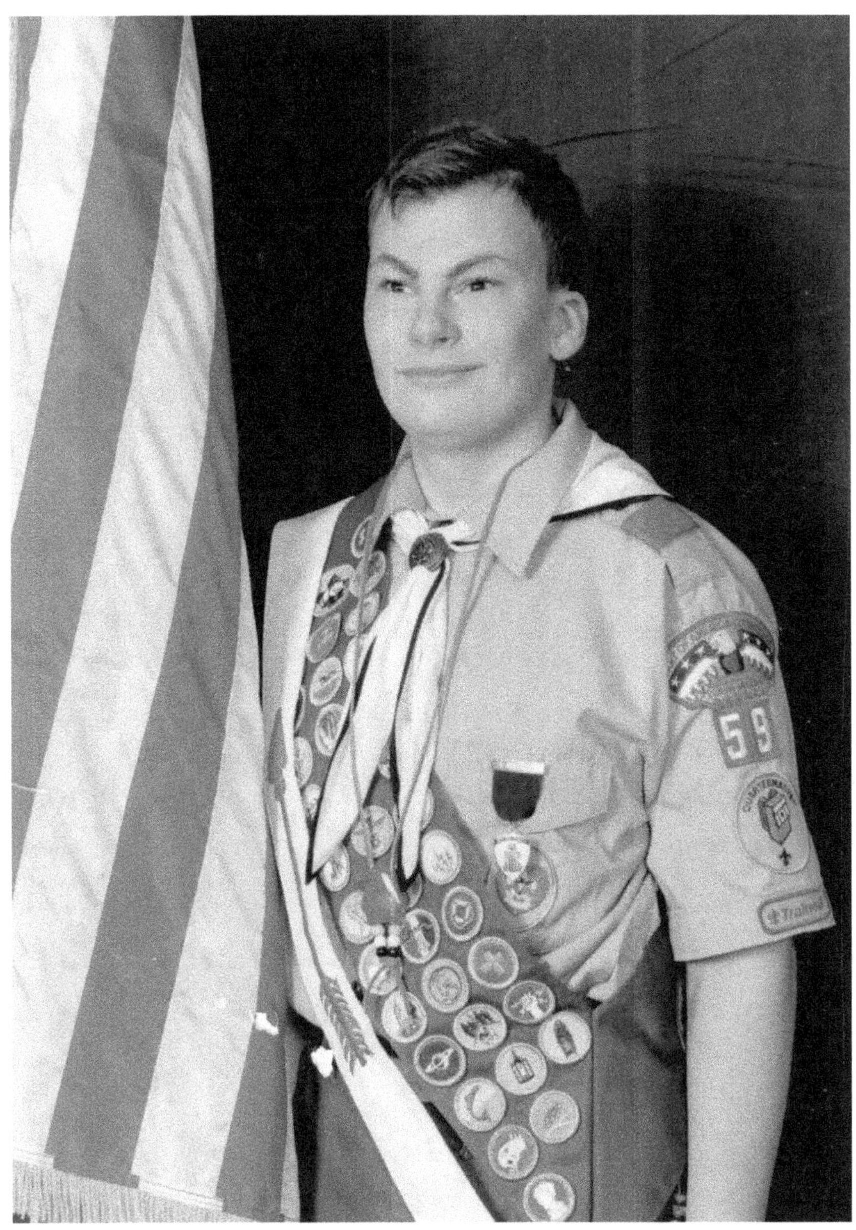

The Eagle Scout

About the Author

Sally Jadlow writes inspirational short stories entitled, *God's Little Miracle Books (I, II, & III);* historical fiction based on fact, *The Late Sooner, The Late Sooner's Daughter,* and *Hard Times in the Heartland;* two 365 day devotionals, *Looking Deeper* and *Daily Walk with Jesus;* a cookbook, *Family Favorites from the Heartland;* and a collection of poetry, *Sonflower Seeds,* all of which are available on Amazon.com.

She resides in Overland Park, Kansas and teaches children and adults the finer points of writing. Sally is also available to speak on many inspirational and writing subjects.

Her blog is located on her website at http://www.SallyJadlow.com.